Beyond the Bowels:

Triumph over Crohn's Challenges

Dr Daniel Harry

Introduction

In the intricate tapestry of human health, certain conditions weave a profound impact on the lives they touch. "Beyond the Bowels: Triumph over Crohn's Challenges" embarks on a journey through the realms of Crohn's disease, offering a comprehensive guide that transcends the physical and delves into the emotional, social, and practical aspects of living with this chronic condition.

Crohn's disease, a form of inflammatory bowel disease (IBD), manifests as more than a mere physiological challenge—it becomes a transformative force reshaping the landscape of daily existence. This book is not merely a compendium of medical facts but a compass for individuals navigating the complexities of Crohn's, helping them chart a course toward understanding, resilience, and triumph.

As we navigate the pages of this book, we will unravel the mystery behind Crohn's, exploring its causes, symptoms, and the intricacies of diagnosis. Beyond the clinical realm, we will delve into the emotional toll exacted by Crohn's, acknowledging the mental fortitude required to face its challenges. Through personal narratives, expert insights, and evidence-based strategies, readers will discover coping mechanisms, support systems, and holistic approaches to managing the disease.

Nutrition, a cornerstone of health, assumes a pivotal role in Crohn's management. This book provides practical guidance on dietary choices, offering a roadmap to nourishment tailored to the unique needs of individuals grappling with the condition. Lifestyle adjustments, encompassing exercise, stress management, and sleep, are explored as essential components of a holistic approach to well-being.

Family, relationships, and the daily intricacies of life are addressed with sensitivity, recognizing the ripple effects that Crohn's can have on these facets. Through stories of resilience and triumph, readers will be inspired to envision a future not defined by limitations but by the unwavering spirit to thrive.

"Beyond the Bowels" is more than a book; it is a companion for those traversing the path of Crohn's, offering guidance, encouragement, and a roadmap to triumph over challenges. Together, let us embark on this journey, transcending the boundaries of the physical ailment and discovering the resilience that resides "Beyond the Bowels."

Chapter 1

Understanding Crohn's

Crohn's disease, a complex and chronic inflammatory condition, significantly impacts the gastrointestinal tract, leading to a myriad of challenges for those affected. In our pursuit of comprehending this intricate ailment, it is essential to grasp the fundamentals that define Crohn's and set the stage for the journey "Beyond the Bowels."

At its core, Crohn's is classified as an inflammatory bowel disease (IBD), a family of disorders that includes ulcerative colitis. Unlike ulcerative colitis, which primarily affects the colon and rectum, Crohn's disease can manifest anywhere along the digestive tract, from the mouth to the anus. This versatility in its presentation makes Crohn's a heterogeneous and often unpredictable condition.

The exact cause of Crohn's remains elusive, but a combination of genetic, environmental, and immune system factors is believed to contribute to its development. Genetic predisposition plays a significant role, as individuals with a family history of IBD are at an increased risk. Environmental factors, such as diet, smoking, and microbial exposures, also influence the likelihood of developing Crohn's.

The hallmark of Crohn's disease lies in the chronic inflammation of the digestive tract. This inflammation can penetrate deep into the layers of the affected tissue, leading to a range of symptoms that vary in severity and presentation. Common symptoms include abdominal pain, diarrhea, weight loss, fatigue, and, in some cases, complications like strictures, abscesses, or fistulas.

Diagnosing Crohn's involves a comprehensive approach, combining clinical evaluation, imaging studies, endoscopic procedures, and laboratory tests. The diagnostic journey is often intricate, requiring a thorough examination to distinguish Crohn's from other gastrointestinal conditions.

While Crohn's primarily affects the gastrointestinal tract, its impact extends far beyond the physical realm. Individuals living with Crohn's often face emotional and social challenges, grappling with the uncertainties of a chronic condition. The unpredictability of symptom flare-ups, coupled with the stigma associated with digestive disorders, can contribute to increased stress and anxiety.

Understanding Crohn's is not merely an academic exercise but a crucial step towards empowering individuals with the knowledge to manage and navigate their journey effectively. In the subsequent chapters of "Beyond the Bowels," we will delve deeper into the intricacies of Crohn's, exploring treatment options, lifestyle adjustments, and the holistic approach required to triumph over its challenges. Through knowledge and resilience, individuals can forge a path towards not just managing but thriving despite Crohn's disease.

The Impact On Quality Of Life

Crohn's disease, with its intricate tapestry of symptoms and uncertainties, extends its influence far beyond the physiological realm, significantly shaping the quality of life for those affected. Understanding the multifaceted impact of Crohn's on daily existence is pivotal in developing strategies for holistic management and fostering resilience.

Chronic Discomfort and Pain:
Living with Crohn's often means contending with persistent abdominal pain and discomfort. The unpredictable nature of flare-ups can disrupt daily activities, making it challenging for individuals to engage fully in work, social events, or even simple

routines. Chronic pain becomes not just a physical burden but a constant companion influencing emotional well-being.

Fatigue and Energy Depletion:
The relentless nature of Crohn's symptoms, coupled with the body's heightened state of alertness during inflammation, frequently leads to chronic fatigue. Individuals may find themselves grappling with a pervasive sense of tiredness, making it difficult to sustain energy levels for work, relationships, and recreational pursuits.

Nutritional Challenges:

The impact of Crohn's on the digestive tract often interferes with proper nutrient absorption, leading to nutritional deficiencies. Dietary restrictions and the fear of triggering symptoms can result in a compromised relationship with food. This, in turn, affects overall well-being and contributes to the physical toll of the disease.

Emotional and Psychological Strain:
The emotional rollercoaster experienced by individuals with Crohn's is profound. Anxiety and depression can surface as they navigate the uncertainties of symptom flare-ups, medical interventions, and the impact on daily life. The

stigma associated with digestive disorders can also contribute to feelings of isolation and reduced self-esteem.

Social Implications:
Crohn's disease can influence social dynamics, as individuals may need to navigate public perceptions, potential embarrassment, or the need for frequent restroom access. Maintaining social connections becomes a delicate balance between managing the condition and fostering meaningful relationships.

Career and Educational Challenges:

The unpredictability of Crohn's symptoms can pose challenges in professional and academic settings. Frequent medical appointments, the need for sick leave during flare-ups, and the impact on concentration and productivity can influence career trajectories and educational pursuits.

Financial Burden:
The economic impact of Crohn's cannot be understated. Medical expenses, including medications, procedures, and potential hospitalizations, can accumulate. Moreover, the potential for work disruptions or limitations may

affect earning capacity, contributing to financial stress.

Understanding and addressing these aspects of Crohn's impact on quality of life requires a holistic approach. Beyond medical interventions, the incorporation of mental health support, nutritional guidance, and strategies for managing the practical challenges of daily life is crucial. In the subsequent chapters of "Beyond the Bowels," we explore avenues to mitigate these challenges, empowering individuals to enhance their quality of life despite the hurdles posed by Crohn's disease.

Unraveling the Basics of Crohn's Disease

Crohn's disease, an enigmatic member of the inflammatory bowel disease (IBD) family, stands as a testament to the complexity of the human body's immune response. As we embark on a journey to unravel the basics of Crohn's, we delve into the intricate mechanisms that underlie this chronic condition. At its essence, Crohn's disease is characterized by chronic inflammation of the gastrointestinal tract, a labyrinthine network extending from the mouth to the anus. Unlike its counterpart, ulcerative colitis, which confines its effects to the colon and rectum, Crohn's exhibits a capricious nature, choosing any segment of the digestive system for its relentless assault.

The origins of Crohn's, while not entirely elucidated, appear to arise from a confluence of genetic predisposition, environmental triggers, and an aberrant immune response. Individuals with a familial history of IBD find themselves at an increased risk, emphasizing the hereditary component of this complex ailment. Environmental factors, ranging from diet to microbial exposures, further complicate the etiological landscape, contributing to the intricate puzzle of why and how Crohn's disease manifests.

Clinically, Crohn's announces its presence through a symphony of symptoms. Abdominal pain, often severe and cramp-like, becomes a persistent companion, accompanied by bouts of diarrhea that may contain blood. Weight loss, fatigue, and a general sense of malaise are common, reflecting the toll that chronic inflammation exacts on the body. The diagnosis of Crohn's is a meticulous process, involving a combination of clinical evaluation, imaging studies, endoscopic procedures, and laboratory tests. Distinguishing Crohn's from other gastrointestinal conditions requires a careful examination of symptoms, paired with a comprehensive understanding of the patient's medical history.

This journey into the basics of Crohn's disease serves as the foundation for a deeper exploration in the chapters that follow. We navigate the complexities of treatment options, unravel the emotional and social dimensions of living with Crohn's, and chart a course toward holistic well-being. As we unravel the mysteries of this condition, the goal remains clear: to empower individuals with the knowledge needed to navigate the challenges posed by Crohn's disease and embark on a path toward resilience and triumph.

Chapter 2

Unraveling The Mystery: Causes And Risk Factors

Crohn's disease, with its intricate origins and complex interplay of factors, stands as a medical enigma, challenging researchers and clinicians alike to decipher the puzzle of its causation. While the precise etiology remains elusive, a convergence of genetic, environmental, and immunological elements contributes to the development of this chronic inflammatory condition.

1. Genetic Predisposition:
One of the cornerstones of Crohn's disease lies in its familial clustering. Individuals with a family history of inflammatory bowel disease (IBD), which includes Crohn's, exhibit a heightened susceptibility. Specific genetic markers, such as variations in the NOD2/CARD15 gene, have been implicated, shedding light on the hereditary component of this intricate puzzle. The interplay of multiple genes likely influences susceptibility, and ongoing research seeks to unravel the intricacies of these genetic factors.

2. Environmental Triggers:

Beyond the genetic tapestry, environmental factors play a pivotal role in triggering or exacerbating Crohn's disease. Dietary habits, notably a high intake of refined sugars and saturated fats, have been associated with an increased risk. Additionally, microbial exposures, including infections and alterations in the gut microbiome, have been explored as potential triggers. The delicate balance between the host and its environment becomes disrupted, unleashing an inflammatory cascade that characterizes Crohn's.

3. Immune System Dysregulation:
At the core of Crohn's pathogenesis lies an aberrant immune response. The immune system, tasked with defending the body against external threats, appears to misinterpret normal gut flora or other environmental factors as intruders, leading to chronic inflammation. Dysregulation in the balance between pro-inflammatory and anti-inflammatory responses contributes to the sustained assault on the gastrointestinal tract, perpetuating the cycle of inflammation seen in Crohn's disease.

4. Genetic-Environmental Interactions:
The interplay between genetic predisposition and environmental triggers unveils the complexity of Crohn's causation. Individuals with a genetic susceptibility may only manifest the disease in the presence of specific environmental factors. This intricate dance between nature and nurture forms the crux of ongoing research endeavors seeking to

identify modifiable risk factors and potential targets for intervention.

As we peel back the layers of Crohn's causation, it becomes evident that no singular factor holds the key to unlocking its mystery. Instead, a web of interactions between genetic, environmental, and immunological elements weaves the intricate narrative of this complex disease. By unraveling these threads, researchers and clinicians strive not only to understand the origins of Crohn's but also to pave the way for personalized therapies and interventions that address the unique factors influencing each individual's journey with this challenging condition.

signs and symptoms: a closer look related to crohn's disease

Crohn's disease, a complex and chronic inflammatory condition, manifests through a spectrum of signs and symptoms that reflect its impact on the gastrointestinal tract. Understanding these clinical manifestations is pivotal for timely diagnosis, effective management, and improving the quality of life for individuals grappling with this multifaceted ailment.

1. Abdominal Pain and Cramping:
Perhaps the most pervasive and characteristic symptom of Crohn's is abdominal pain. The pain is often localized to the lower right side of the abdomen, but its intensity and location can vary. Cramp-like sensations accompany this pain, with severity ranging from mild discomfort to debilitating spasms. The unpredictable nature of these abdominal pains can significantly disrupt daily activities and contribute to the overall burden of the disease.

2. Diarrhea:
Chronic diarrhea, sometimes with urgency, is a hallmark feature of Crohn's disease. The inflammation and ulceration of the gastrointestinal tract disrupt the normal absorption of water and nutrients, leading to loose and frequent bowel movements. The presence of blood in the stool is not uncommon, indicating the extent of inflammation and potential ulceration within the digestive tract.

3. Weight Loss and Malnutrition:
The chronic nature of Crohn's, coupled with symptoms like diarrhea and malabsorption, often leads to weight loss. Nutrient deficiencies may arise due to impaired absorption in the inflamed intestine, contributing to malnutrition. Individuals with Crohn's

may experience a decline in muscle mass and overall energy levels, further impacting their quality of life.

4. Fatigue:
The relentless nature of Crohn's symptoms, coupled with the body's heightened state of alertness during inflammation, frequently leads to chronic fatigue. Individuals may find themselves grappling with a pervasive sense of tiredness, making it challenging to sustain energy levels for work, relationships, and recreational pursuits.

5. Fever and Systemic Symptoms:
In severe cases, Crohn's disease can induce systemic symptoms, including fever. This may indicate complications such as abscess formation or the body's heightened inflammatory response. Systemic symptoms, coupled with localized abdominal pain, underscore the dynamic nature of Crohn's and its potential to affect the entire body.

6. Extraintestinal Manifestations:
Crohn's is not confined solely to the gastrointestinal tract; it can also manifest in extraintestinal areas. Joint pain, skin rashes, and eye inflammation are among the extraintestinal manifestations associated with Crohn's. These symptoms further underscore the systemic impact of the disease and highlight the need for a comprehensive approach to its management.

7. Perianal Symptoms:
In some cases, Crohn's disease can lead to perianal complications such as fistulas (abnormal connections between organs), abscesses, or fissures. These symptoms add an additional layer of complexity to the disease and may require specific interventions for effective management.

Understanding the nuanced interplay of these signs and symptoms is crucial for healthcare providers in diagnosing Crohn's disease. Additionally, for individuals living with Crohn's, recognizing these manifestations allows for proactive management and enhances communication with healthcare professionals. The journey "Beyond the Bowels" involves not just understanding these symptoms but navigating their impact on daily life and forging a path toward effective management and resilience.

Diagnosis And Differentiating Factors Related To Crohn's Disease

The diagnostic journey for Crohn's disease is a meticulous process that involves a combination of clinical evaluation, imaging studies, endoscopic procedures, and laboratory tests. Distinguishing Crohn's from other gastrointestinal conditions requires a thorough understanding of the presenting symptoms, coupled with a nuanced examination of the patient's medical history. Here, we delve into the intricacies of the diagnostic process and explore the differentiating factors that guide healthcare professionals in accurately identifying Crohn's disease.

1. Clinical Evaluation:
The diagnostic process typically begins with a detailed clinical evaluation. Healthcare providers collect a comprehensive medical history, including information about symptoms, their duration, and any relevant family history of inflammatory bowel disease (IBD). Understanding the patient's overall

health, lifestyle, and potential triggers for symptoms contributes to the initial assessment.

2. Physical Examination:
A thorough physical examination complements the clinical evaluation. Abdominal tenderness, palpable masses, or signs of nutritional deficiencies may be evident during the examination. Extra-intestinal manifestations, such as joint pain or skin abnormalities, may also be assessed.

3. Laboratory Tests:
Blood tests play a crucial role in the diagnostic process. Elevated levels of inflammatory markers, such as C-reactive protein (CRP) and erythrocyte sedimentation rate (ESR), are indicative of an inflammatory process. Anemia, often associated with chronic inflammation, may also be detected. Additionally, blood tests can assess for nutritional deficiencies, such as low levels of iron, vitamin B12, or vitamin D.

4. Imaging Studies:
Various imaging modalities aid in visualizing the gastrointestinal tract and identifying signs of inflammation or complications. Abdominal imaging, including computed tomography (CT) scans or magnetic resonance imaging (MRI), provides detailed views of the intestines. These imaging studies help evaluate the extent and severity of inflammation and identify potential complications such as strictures or abscesses.

5. Endoscopic Procedures:

Endoscopy is a cornerstone in the diagnosis of Crohn's disease. Colonoscopy and upper endoscopy (esophagogastroduodenoscopy or EGD) allow direct visualization of the intestinal lining. During these procedures, healthcare providers can obtain biopsies for histological examination, aiding in confirming the presence of inflammation and ruling out other conditions.

6. Differentiating Factors:

Distinguishing Crohn's from other gastrointestinal conditions, particularly ulcerative colitis, is crucial. While both are forms of inflammatory bowel disease, they have distinct characteristics. Crohn's can affect any part of the digestive tract, while ulcerative colitis is limited to the colon and rectum. The pattern of inflammation in Crohn's, often characterized by skip lesions and transmural involvement, differs from the continuous and superficial inflammation seen in ulcerative colitis.

7. Rule-Out Process:

The diagnostic process for Crohn's also involves ruling out other conditions that may present with similar symptoms. Conditions such as irritable bowel syndrome (IBS), celiac disease, and infections must be considered and excluded through appropriate tests.

The journey to a conclusive diagnosis of Crohn's disease requires a collaborative effort between healthcare providers and individuals experiencing symptoms. The integration of clinical evaluation, laboratory tests, imaging studies, and endoscopic procedures allows for a comprehensive understanding of the disease's characteristics and aids in formulating an effective management plan. A precise diagnosis serves as the foundation for navigating the complexities of Crohn's and embarking on a path toward tailored treatment and improved quality of life.

crohn's journey begins

The initiation of the Crohn's journey marks the commencement of an odyssey into the intricate and often challenging landscape of living with a chronic condition. As individuals find themselves at the crossroads of diagnosis, the realization dawns that Crohn's disease transcends mere medical nomenclature; it becomes a defining aspect of daily existence. This section of the journey signifies the onset of a dynamic relationship with treatment modalities, lifestyle adjustments, and the continuous ebb and flow of symptoms. Navigating this complex terrain requires resilience, adaptability, and a holistic approach to well-being. From exploring the myriad treatment options, understanding the role of medications and surgical interventions, to embracing the nuances of dietary and lifestyle adjustments, individuals with Crohn's embark on a path uniquely their own. This is not merely a clinical expedition; it is a personal odyssey, marked by triumphs, setbacks, and a continual quest for balance. As the Crohn's journey begins, so too does the pursuit of empowerment, knowledge, and the unwavering spirit to thrive despite the challenges posed by this chronic and unpredictable condition. Through the pages that follow, we delve into the multifaceted aspects of this journey, offering insights, strategies, and narratives that illuminate the path toward not just managing but triumphing over the complexities of Crohn's disease.

Chapter 3

Navigating Treatment Options

The management of Crohn's disease involves a nuanced and personalized approach, considering the varied symptoms and individual responses to treatment. As we navigate the complex landscape of therapeutic interventions, it becomes evident that no one-size-fits-all solution exists for this chronic condition. The treatment journey is marked by a continuous assessment of symptoms, the pursuit of remission, and the mitigation of complications. Here, we delve into the diverse array of treatment options available for individuals with Crohn's disease, recognizing the importance of a multidisciplinary approach to achieve optimal outcomes.

1. Medications:
Medications play a central role in the management of Crohn's disease, aiming to control inflammation and alleviate symptoms. A spectrum of options includes aminosalicylates, corticosteroids, immunomodulators, and biologics. The choice of medication depends on the severity of symptoms, the location of inflammation, and individual responses. Biologics, such as anti-tumor necrosis factor (TNF) agents, represent a significant advancement, offering targeted therapies to modulate the immune response.

2. Nutritional Therapy:
Nutritional interventions are integral to Crohn's management, addressing not only symptom relief but also promoting overall well-being. Exclusive enteral nutrition (EEN), involving liquid nutrition as the sole source of nourishment, has shown efficacy, particularly in pediatric cases. Additionally, dietary modifications, such as low-residue or low-FODMAP diets, are explored to manage specific symptoms and improve nutritional status.

3. Surgical Interventions:
Surgery becomes a consideration when medications are unable to control symptoms or when complications arise. Common surgical procedures include the removal of diseased portions of the intestine, strictureplasty to widen narrowed segments, or the creation of ostomies in cases of severe disease. Surgical interventions aim

to alleviate symptoms, correct complications, and improve overall quality of life.

4. Lifestyle Adjustments:
Lifestyle modifications are crucial components of Crohn's management. Regular exercise, stress management, and adequate sleep contribute to overall well-being. However, it's essential to tailor these adjustments to individual capabilities and take into account the potential impact on symptoms.

5. Integrative Approaches:
Complementary and integrative therapies, such as acupuncture, probiotics, and mind-body techniques, are explored for their potential to enhance symptom management and improve quality of life. While evidence varies for these approaches, some individuals find value in incorporating them into their overall care plan.

6. Patient-Centered Decision-Making:
The complexity of Crohn's treatment necessitates a patient-centered approach, emphasizing shared decision-making between individuals and healthcare providers. Understanding treatment options, potential risks, and benefits empowers individuals to actively participate in shaping their care plan.

7. Ongoing Monitoring and Adjustments:

Crohn's is a dynamic condition, and treatment plans require continual assessment and adjustments. Regular follow-ups, monitoring of symptoms, and objective markers such as inflammatory markers or imaging studies guide healthcare providers in modifying treatment strategies as needed.

As we navigate the diverse array of treatment options, the journey with Crohn's becomes a collaborative effort, marked by open communication, adaptability, and a commitment to enhancing the overall quality of life. Recognizing the individuality of each person's experience, the treatment approach seeks not just to manage symptoms but to empower individuals to thrive in the face of Crohn's disease.

Medications And Their Roles

The pharmacological management of Crohn's disease is a dynamic and evolving landscape, marked by a diverse array of medications aimed at controlling inflammation, alleviating symptoms, and achieving sustained remission. As we explore the roles of these medications, it becomes clear that the choice and combination of drugs depend on factors such as disease severity, location, and the individual's response. Here, we delve into the various classes of medications commonly employed in the treatment of Crohn's, shedding light on their mechanisms, benefits, and considerations.

1. Aminosalicylates:
Aminosalicylates, including drugs such as mesalamine, sulfasalazine, and olsalazine, are often used in the management of mild to moderate Crohn's disease, particularly in cases where inflammation is limited to the colon. These medications have anti-inflammatory properties and are commonly administered orally or rectally to target localized inflammation.

2. Corticosteroids:
Corticosteroids, such as prednisone and budesonide, are potent anti-inflammatory agents employed for short-term relief of moderate to

severe symptoms during disease flares. However, their long-term use is limited due to potential side effects, including bone density loss, weight gain, and immunosuppression.

3. Immunomodulators:
Immunomodulators, including azathioprine, mercaptopurine, and methotrexate, act on the immune system to modulate its response. These medications are often considered for individuals with moderate to severe disease or those who do not respond to aminosalicylates or corticosteroids. Immunomodulators may take weeks to months to achieve therapeutic effects.

4. Biologics:
Biologics represent a groundbreaking class of medications designed to target specific components of the immune system implicated in Crohn's disease. Anti-tumor necrosis factor (TNF) agents, such as infliximab, adalimumab, and certolizumab pegol, are widely used to induce and maintain remission in moderate to severe cases. Other biologics, including vedolizumab and ustekinumab, target different pathways in the immune response.

5. Janus Kinase (JAK) Inhibitors:
JAK inhibitors, such as tofacitinib, are oral medications that modulate the immune response. They are employed in cases where other medications may be ineffective or poorly tolerated.

JAK inhibitors offer an additional option for achieving and maintaining remission.

6. Antibiotics:
Antibiotics, such as metronidazole and ciprofloxacin, are sometimes used to address infections or complications associated with Crohn's disease, particularly in cases of perianal involvement or fistulas. They are not typically used as primary maintenance therapy.

7. Topical Therapies:
Rectal therapies, including corticosteroid or mesalamine enemas or suppositories, are used to target inflammation in the rectum and lower portions of the colon. These topical treatments are particularly valuable in cases of localized disease or for individuals who have difficulty tolerating oral medications.

Considerations and Individualized Approaches:
The selection of medications for Crohn's disease necessitates careful consideration of individual factors, including disease phenotype, comorbidities, and the presence of complications. Additionally, the potential for side effects and the individual's preferences and lifestyle play a crucial role in crafting an effective and sustainable treatment plan.

In the dynamic landscape of Crohn's disease management, medication choices are continually evolving. The goal remains to achieve sustained remission, alleviate symptoms, and improve the overall quality of life. Collaborative discussions between healthcare providers and individuals with Crohn's empower informed decision-making, ensuring that the chosen medications align with the unique needs and goals of each person on their journey with Crohn's disease.

Surgical Interventions:

Surgical interventions play a significant role in the management of Crohn's disease, addressing complications, improving quality of life, and, in some cases, offering a respite from debilitating symptoms. Understanding the rationale behind surgical procedures, the potential outcomes, and what to expect during the preoperative and postoperative phases is crucial for individuals navigating the complexities of Crohn's disease.

1. Indications for Surgery:
Surgical intervention in Crohn's disease is often prompted by specific indications, including the failure of medical management, the presence of complications, or the need to address symptoms that significantly impact daily life. Common indications include bowel strictures, fistulas, abscesses, and refractory disease not responsive to medications.

2. Bowel Resection:
Bowel resection is a common surgical procedure for individuals with Crohn's disease, particularly when strictures or localized inflammation affect a segment of the intestine. The surgeon removes the diseased portion of the bowel, aiming to alleviate symptoms, improve function, and prevent complications.

3. Strictureplasty:
In cases where multiple segments of the intestine are affected by strictures, strictureplasty may be performed. This technique involves widening the narrowed portions of the bowel without removing them, preserving as much healthy tissue as possible.

4. Fistula Repair:
Fistulas, abnormal connections between organs or tissues, are another complication of Crohn's disease. Surgical intervention may be necessary to

repair or redirect these fistulas, addressing the associated pain, infection, and other symptoms.

5. Abscess Drainage:
Abscesses, pockets of infection, can develop in individuals with Crohn's disease. Surgical drainage may be required to remove the accumulated pus and prevent the spread of infection.

6. Ostomy Creation:
In severe cases where extensive disease or complications necessitate the diversion of stool away from the affected area, the creation of an ostomy may be considered. This can involve the formation of an ileostomy or colostomy, providing an alternative route for waste elimination.

Preoperative Considerations:
Before surgery, individuals with Crohn's disease undergo a thorough preoperative assessment. This involves medical evaluations, imaging studies, and discussions about the surgical plan, potential complications, and expected outcomes. Nutritional support may be initiated to optimize the individual's overall health.

Postoperative Recovery:
Postoperative recovery varies depending on the nature and extent of the surgery. Individuals can expect a period of hospitalization, followed by a gradual return to regular activities. Pain management, nutritional support, and monitoring

for potential complications, such as infections or bowel obstructions, are integral components of the postoperative care plan.

Managing Expectations:
While surgical interventions can provide significant relief and improve overall well-being, it's important to acknowledge that Crohn's disease is a chronic condition, and surgery does not constitute a cure. Individuals may experience periods of remission, but ongoing medical management and regular follow-ups remain crucial to address potential disease recurrence or complications.

Psychosocial Support:
The psychosocial impact of surgery on individuals with Crohn's disease is substantial. Support from healthcare professionals, mental health specialists, and peer support groups is essential in navigating the emotional aspects of surgery, including concerns about body image, lifestyle adjustments, and the impact on relationships.

In navigating the landscape of surgical interventions for Crohn's disease, a collaborative approach between individuals, healthcare providers, and a multidisciplinary care team is paramount. Clear communication, informed decision-making, and ongoing support contribute to a holistic strategy for managing Crohn's, encompassing both medical and surgical aspects, with the ultimate goal of enhancing quality of life and fostering resilience on the journey "Beyond the Bowels."

Beyond The Physical: The Emotional Toll

The narrative of Crohn's disease extends far beyond the tangible symptoms and medical interventions, weaving a profound emotional tapestry that shapes the lived experience of those affected. As individuals embark on the intricate journey of managing Crohn's, they traverse not only the physical challenges but also the intricate terrain of emotional resilience. The emotional toll exacted by this chronic condition is palpable—the uncertainty of flare-ups, the relentless nature of symptoms, and the impact on daily life all contribute to a complex emotional landscape. Anxiety and depression often find a foothold as individuals grapple with the unpredictability of their condition. The stigma associated with digestive disorders can cast shadows on self-esteem, and the constant need for adaptation can evoke feelings of frustration and weariness. Yet, within this emotional labyrinth, stories of courage, perseverance, and resilience emerge. This section delves into the multifaceted dimensions of the emotional toll associated with Crohn's, acknowledging the challenges while illuminating avenues for support, coping, and finding strength in the face of adversity. Through shared narratives, expert insights, and strategies for emotional well-being, we unravel the threads that connect the physical and emotional aspects of Crohn's disease, recognizing that the journey "Beyond the Bowels" encompasses not only the management of symptoms but also the cultivation of a resilient spirit that thrives despite the emotional complexities woven into the fabric of this chronic condition.

Chapter 4

Coping With The Mental And Emotional Challenges

The emotional landscape of Crohn's disease is intricate, marked by the ebb and flow of symptoms, the unpredictability of flare-ups, and the pervasive impact on daily life. Coping with the mental and emotional challenges associated with this chronic condition requires a nuanced and holistic approach, acknowledging the interplay between physical health and emotional well-being. Here, we explore strategies, insights, and narratives that shed light on navigating the emotional complexities of Crohn's, empowering individuals to not only manage the physical aspects of the disease but also foster resilience in the face of mental and emotional challenges.

1. Building a Supportive Network:
Establishing a robust support network is foundational in coping with the emotional challenges of Crohn's. Family, friends, and peers who understand the nuances of the condition provide not only practical assistance but also invaluable emotional support. Online communities and support groups offer spaces for individuals to share experiences, gain insights, and foster a sense of belonging.

2. Open Communication with Healthcare Providers:

Transparent communication with healthcare providers is pivotal in addressing emotional challenges. Sharing concerns, fears, and the emotional impact of the disease enables a collaborative approach to care. Healthcare professionals can offer guidance on mental health resources, coping strategies, and potential adjustments to the treatment plan to enhance overall well-being.

3. Mind-Body Techniques:
Incorporating mind-body techniques, such as mindfulness meditation, deep breathing exercises, or yoga, can be transformative in managing stress and promoting emotional balance. These practices not only provide a respite from the emotional toll but also contribute to overall mental well-being.

4. Counseling and Therapy:
Seeking professional counseling or therapy is a proactive step in addressing the emotional challenges of Crohn's. Mental health professionals can offer coping strategies, tools for managing anxiety or depression, and a safe space for individuals to explore and process the emotional impact of the disease.

5. Education and Empowerment:
Understanding the intricacies of Crohn's disease fosters a sense of empowerment. Education about the condition, treatment options, and potential challenges equips individuals with the knowledge needed to navigate the journey effectively. Empowerment through knowledge reduces the sense of uncertainty and enhances one's ability to advocate for their own well-being.

6. Artistic Expression and Creativity:
Engaging in artistic expression, whether through writing, art, or music, can serve as a therapeutic outlet for emotions. Creative pursuits provide a means of self-expression, allowing individuals to channel their experiences and emotions into a tangible form.

7. Setting Realistic Goals:
Setting realistic goals and expectations is crucial in mitigating the emotional impact of Crohn's. Recognizing and celebrating small achievements, adjusting expectations during flare-ups, and practicing self-compassion contribute to a positive mindset.

8. Social Connection:
Despite the challenges, maintaining social connections is vital for emotional well-being. Balancing social activities with self-care, communicating openly with friends and loved ones,

and fostering a sense of normalcy contribute to a supportive social environment.

9. Addressing Stigma:

Confronting and addressing the stigma associated with Crohn's is an integral aspect of coping emotionally. Advocating for awareness, educating others about the condition, and fostering a supportive community contribute to dismantling stereotypes and reducing the emotional burden associated with stigma.

Navigating the mental and emotional challenges of Crohn's disease is a dynamic process, and individuals often find a combination of these strategies most effective. Recognizing that emotional well-being is a crucial component of overall health, the journey "Beyond the Bowels" encompasses not only the management of physical symptoms but also the cultivation of resilience, emotional strength, and a thriving spirit despite the challenges posed by Crohn's disease.

Building A Support System

The journey with Crohn's disease is inherently challenging, requiring not only medical management but also a robust support system to navigate the emotional and practical complexities. Building and maintaining a strong support network is paramount for individuals grappling with the impact of this chronic condition. From family and friends to healthcare providers and peer communities, a well-constructed support system becomes a pillar of strength, fostering resilience and empowerment. Here, we explore the elements of a comprehensive support system for individuals living with Crohn's disease, offering insights, strategies, and narratives that illuminate the path to thriving beyond the physical challenges.

1. Family and Friends:
The foundational layer of a support system often comprises family and friends. Open and honest communication with loved ones is essential, helping

them understand the nuances of Crohn's and fostering empathy. Family and friends can provide practical assistance, emotional support, and a sense of connection during both the highs and lows of the disease.

2. Healthcare Providers:

Establishing a collaborative relationship with healthcare providers is crucial in building a support system. Regular communication, transparent discussions about symptoms and concerns, and a shared decision-making approach empower individuals to actively participate in their care. Healthcare providers offer not only medical expertise but also guidance on mental health resources and strategies for overall well-being.

3. Support Groups and Peer Communities:
Joining support groups and peer communities tailored to individuals with Crohn's disease provides a unique space for shared experiences and understanding. Online forums, local meet-ups, and organized support groups offer avenues to connect, exchange insights, and gain emotional support from those who navigate similar challenges.

4. Counseling and Therapy:
Professional counseling or therapy is a valuable component of a comprehensive support system.

Mental health professionals can offer coping strategies, tools for managing stress, and a safe environment for individuals to explore and process the emotional impact of Crohn's.

5. Patient Advocacy Organizations:
Patient advocacy organizations dedicated to Crohn's disease play a pivotal role in offering resources, educational materials, and community engagement opportunities. These organizations often host events, provide access to expert insights, and advocate for the needs of individuals with Crohn's on a broader scale.

6. Educational Workshops and Webinars:
Attending educational workshops and webinars focused on Crohn's disease provides not only valuable information but also opportunities to connect with others facing similar challenges. These events often cover a range of topics, from treatment options to lifestyle adjustments, fostering a sense of empowerment through knowledge.

7. Online Platforms and Social Media:
Utilizing online platforms and social media for support and information exchange can be a dynamic aspect of a support system. Engaging with reputable websites, forums, and social media groups allows individuals to access a wealth of shared experiences, tips, and updates related to Crohn's disease.

8. Self-Help Strategies:
Encouraging the development of self-help strategies within the support system empowers individuals to actively contribute to their well-being. This may include setting personal goals, practicing stress-reduction techniques, and incorporating hobbies or activities that bring joy and fulfillment.

9. Caregiver Support:
Acknowledging and addressing the needs of caregivers is an integral part of a holistic support system. Caregiver support groups, resources, and open communication between individuals with Crohn's and their caregivers foster a collaborative and understanding environment.

10. Advocacy and Awareness:
Engaging in advocacy and awareness initiatives can contribute to building a supportive community not only for oneself but for others affected by Crohn's. By sharing personal experiences, participating in awareness campaigns, and fostering understanding, individuals become advocates for positive change.

Building a robust support system for thriving with Crohn's disease is a dynamic and ongoing process. Recognizing that the journey "Beyond the Bowels" encompasses not only medical management but also emotional well-being, a comprehensive support system serves as a vital foundation for resilience, empowerment, and a thriving life despite the challenges posed by Crohn's disease.

Mental Health Strategies

The intricate interplay between physical health and mental well-being in the context of Crohn's disease necessitates a holistic approach to overall health. Individuals grappling with the complexities of this chronic condition often find that mental health strategies play a pivotal role in managing not only the emotional challenges but also the impact on daily life. From stress management to cultivating resilience, the following comprehensive guide explores a spectrum of mental health strategies tailored to individuals navigating the unique landscape of Crohn's disease.

1. Mindfulness and Meditation:
Incorporating mindfulness practices and meditation techniques provides individuals with Crohn's a

powerful tool for managing stress and promoting emotional balance. Mindful breathing, guided meditation, or mindfulness-based stress reduction (MBSR) can be practiced regularly to cultivate a sense of calm and enhance overall mental well-being.

2. Stress Reduction Techniques:
Chronic stress can exacerbate symptoms of Crohn's disease. Implementing stress reduction techniques, such as deep breathing exercises, progressive muscle relaxation, or engaging in activities that bring joy and relaxation, can contribute to a more resilient response to stressors.

3. Cognitive Behavioral Therapy (CBT):
CBT is a therapeutic approach that focuses on identifying and modifying negative thought patterns and behaviors. It can be particularly beneficial for individuals with Crohn's in addressing anxiety, depression, and coping with the emotional impact of the disease.

4. Regular Physical Activity:
Exercise has been shown to have positive effects on both physical and mental well-being. Engaging in regular physical activity not only supports overall health but also contributes to stress reduction and the release of endorphins, promoting a more positive mood.

5. Nutrition and Gut-Brain Connection:

Recognizing the connection between gut health and mental well-being, individuals with Crohn's can explore nutrition strategies that support both aspects. A balanced diet, rich in nutrients and tailored to individual tolerances, contributes not only to physical health but also to emotional resilience.

6. Sleep Hygiene:
Adequate and quality sleep is integral to mental health. Establishing good sleep hygiene practices, such as maintaining a consistent sleep schedule, creating a comfortable sleep environment, and avoiding stimulants before bedtime, supports overall well-being.

7. Social Connection:
Cultivating social connections is a powerful mental health strategy. Whether through in-person interactions or virtual communities, maintaining meaningful relationships reduces feelings of isolation, fosters support, and provides a sense of belonging.

8. Journaling and Self-Reflection:
Journaling allows individuals to express their thoughts, emotions, and experiences. Reflecting on daily experiences, challenges, and victories provides a therapeutic outlet for processing emotions and gaining insights into one's mental and emotional landscape.

9. Setting Realistic Goals:
Setting realistic and achievable goals, both short-term and long-term, contributes to a sense of accomplishment and boosts self-esteem. Breaking down larger tasks into smaller, manageable steps allows for a proactive and positive approach to daily challenges.

10. Professional Mental Health Support:
Seeking professional mental health support, such as counseling or therapy, is a proactive step in addressing the emotional challenges associated with Crohn's. Mental health professionals provide tools for coping, strategies for stress management, and a safe space for exploring and processing emotions.

11. Educational Empowerment:
Empowering oneself through education about Crohn's disease and mental health fosters a sense of control and understanding. Knowing about the condition, treatment options, and potential challenges contributes to a more informed and empowered approach to managing both physical and mental health.

12. Mind-Body Practices:
Engaging in mind-body practices, such as yoga or tai chi, integrates physical movement with mindfulness, promoting relaxation and overall mental well-being. These practices offer a holistic

approach that addresses both physical and emotional aspects.

In navigating the mental health strategies associated with Crohn's disease, individuals may find a combination of these approaches most effective. Recognizing that mental well-being is a dynamic and individualized aspect of overall health, the journey "Beyond the Bowels" encompasses not only medical management but also the cultivation of resilience, emotional strength, and a thriving spirit despite the challenges posed by Crohn's disease.

Diet And Nutrition In Crohn's

In the intricate tapestry of Crohn's disease management, the significance of diet and nutrition emerges as a cornerstone for achieving balance and well-being. This chronic inflammatory condition places unique demands on the digestive system, prompting individuals to navigate a complex relationship between food choices and symptom management. The journey "Beyond the Bowels" requires a nuanced understanding of how dietary strategies can contribute to both physical health and emotional resilience. From identifying trigger foods to embracing nutritional support, this section delves into the intricate interplay of diet and Crohn's management. It explores not only the practical aspects of crafting a diet tailored to individual needs but also the emotional resilience cultivated through informed choices. Through a comprehensive exploration of dietary considerations, nutritional therapies, and the art of finding harmony between nourishment and symptom alleviation, individuals with Crohn's are empowered to embark on a journey of self-discovery, where the choices on their plate become integral threads in the fabric of well-being.

Chapter 5

The Role Of Diet In Crohn's Disease

Diet plays a pivotal role in the intricate management of Crohn's disease, a chronic inflammatory condition affecting the gastrointestinal tract. The complex interplay between diet and Crohn's involves not only identifying trigger foods that may exacerbate symptoms but also exploring nutritional strategies to support overall well-being. Recognizing that dietary needs can vary among individuals, a tailored approach is crucial. Here, we delve into the multifaceted role of diet in Crohn's management, exploring considerations ranging from symptom alleviation to nutritional support and the cultivation of a balanced and resilient lifestyle.

1. Identifying Trigger Foods:
For individuals with Crohn's, certain foods may trigger or worsen symptoms during flare-ups. Common triggers include high-fiber foods, dairy products, spicy foods, and certain raw fruits and vegetables. Keeping a food diary and working closely with healthcare providers and nutritionists can help identify and manage these triggers, allowing for a more individualized dietary approach.

2. Low-Residue and Low-FODMAP Diets:

Low-residue and low-FODMAP (fermentable oligosaccharides, disaccharides, monosaccharides, and polyols) diets are often explored to manage symptoms in individuals with Crohn's. These dietary approaches involve minimizing the intake of certain carbohydrates and fibers that can be challenging to digest, potentially reducing symptoms such as bloating, gas, and abdominal discomfort.

3. Nutritional Support During Flare-Ups:
During flare-ups, individuals with Crohn's may experience reduced appetite, weight loss, and nutritional deficiencies. Nutritional support, including liquid diets, nutritional supplements, and, in some cases, exclusive enteral nutrition (EEN), can provide essential nutrients and promote healing while giving the digestive system a temporary respite.

4. Individualized Nutrient Assessment:
Crohn's disease can impact the absorption of nutrients, leading to deficiencies. Regular assessments of nutritional status, including levels of vitamins and minerals, are essential. Individualized supplementation may be recommended to address deficiencies and support overall health.

5. Gradual Introduction of Foods:
After periods of symptom management or following surgical interventions, a gradual reintroduction of

foods is often recommended. This step-by-step approach allows individuals to identify tolerances and preferences while minimizing the risk of triggering symptoms.

6. Protein-Rich and Nutrient-Dense Foods:
Protein-rich and nutrient-dense foods play a crucial role in supporting overall health for individuals with Crohn's. Lean proteins, such as poultry, fish, and eggs, along with nutrient-dense fruits, vegetables, and whole grains that are well-tolerated, contribute essential vitamins and minerals.

7. Hydration and Fluid Balance:
Maintaining adequate hydration is paramount, especially during flare-ups when there may be increased fluid losses. Monitoring fluid intake and adjusting based on individual needs help support hydration and prevent complications related to dehydration.

8. Collaboration with Healthcare Providers:
Collaboration with healthcare providers, including gastroenterologists, dietitians, and nutritionists, is fundamental. A team approach ensures that dietary recommendations align with medical management, addressing both the nutritional needs and symptom management goals of individuals with Crohn's.

9. Lifestyle Considerations:
Beyond specific dietary choices, lifestyle considerations, such as regular physical activity,

stress management, and adequate sleep, contribute to overall well-being. These factors play an interconnected role in managing Crohn's and promoting a balanced and resilient lifestyle.

10. Ongoing Adaptation and Monitoring:
The dynamic nature of Crohn's disease requires ongoing adaptation of dietary strategies. Regular monitoring of symptoms, nutritional status, and discussions with healthcare providers allow for adjustments to the dietary approach as needed.

Navigating Crohn's disease through diet involves a

thoughtful and individualized approach. By understanding the intricate relationship between food choices and symptoms, individuals can craft a dietary strategy that aligns with their unique needs and empowers them to actively manage their condition while fostering a sense of balance and resilience in their journey "Beyond the Bowels."

nutritional approaches for better health related to crohn's disease

Nutrition stands as a cornerstone in the holistic management of Crohn's disease, a chronic inflammatory condition with unique challenges centered around the gastrointestinal tract. A thoughtful and individualized nutritional approach can significantly impact the well-being of individuals navigating this complex condition. From identifying trigger foods to optimizing nutrient intake, the following exploration delves into comprehensive nutritional strategies designed to promote better health, manage symptoms, and support resilience for those embracing the journey "Beyond the Bowels."

1. Individualized Nutrition Plans:
Recognizing the highly individual nature of Crohn's disease, personalized nutrition plans are fundamental. Collaborating with healthcare providers, particularly registered dietitians specializing in gastrointestinal disorders, allows for the development of plans tailored to individual needs, taking into account triggers, tolerances, and nutritional goals.

2. Balanced Macronutrient Intake:
Achieving a balance in macronutrient intake—proteins, fats, and carbohydrates—is vital for

individuals with Crohn's. Focusing on lean proteins, healthy fats, and well-tolerated carbohydrates contributes to sustained energy levels and overall nutritional well-being.

3. Optimizing Micronutrient Intake:
Crohn's disease can impact the absorption of essential vitamins and minerals. A focus on optimizing micronutrient intake through a variety of nutrient-dense foods and, when necessary, supplementation, helps prevent deficiencies and supports overall health.

4. Omega-3 Fatty Acids:
Omega-3 fatty acids, found in fatty fish such as salmon and flaxseeds, exhibit anti-inflammatory properties. Incorporating these into the diet may contribute to managing inflammation associated with Crohn's disease. However, individual tolerances should be considered.

5. Probiotics and Gut Health:
Probiotics, beneficial bacteria that support gut health, are explored by some individuals with Crohn's to promote a balanced microbiome. While research on their efficacy is ongoing, discussing probiotic use with healthcare providers is essential to ensure safety and appropriateness for individual cases.

6. Hydration and Electrolyte Balance:

Maintaining adequate hydration is crucial, particularly during flare-ups when there may be increased fluid losses. Emphasizing electrolyte-rich foods and beverages, such as bananas or electrolyte solutions, supports hydration and helps prevent complications related to dehydration.

7. Prebiotics and Fiber:
While high-fiber foods can be challenging for some individuals with Crohn's, prebiotic-rich foods may support a healthy gut microbiome. Gradual introduction of well-tolerated sources, such as bananas, garlic, and asparagus, allows for the potential benefits of prebiotics without exacerbating symptoms.

8. Consideration of Food Sensitivities:
Identifying and addressing food sensitivities is integral. Some individuals may benefit from elimination diets or targeted exclusion of specific trigger foods identified through close monitoring and collaboration with healthcare providers.

9. Anti-Inflammatory Foods:
Incorporating anti-inflammatory foods, such as turmeric, ginger, and green leafy vegetables, may contribute to managing inflammation associated with Crohn's disease. While these foods may offer potential benefits, individual tolerances should be considered.

10. Supplemental Nutrition:

In cases of malnutrition, weight loss, or during flare-ups, supplemental nutrition may be necessary. This can include liquid nutritional supplements, enteral nutrition, or, in severe cases, parenteral nutrition administered intravenously under medical supervision.

11. Consultation with Healthcare Providers:
Regular consultation with healthcare providers is crucial for ongoing nutritional management. Open communication allows for adjustments to nutrition plans based on changes in symptoms, disease activity, or overall health status.

12. Emphasis on Overall Well-Being:
Beyond specific nutritional considerations, emphasizing overall well-being through a balanced lifestyle is essential. This includes regular physical activity, stress management, and adequate sleep—all contributing factors to a comprehensive approach to health.

Navigating Crohn's disease through nutritional approaches requires adaptability and ongoing collaboration with healthcare providers. By integrating these strategies into daily life, individuals can actively contribute to their overall well-being, manage symptoms effectively, and embark on a journey "Beyond the Bowels" that encompasses not only physical health but also resilience and a thriving spirit despite the challenges posed by Crohn's disease.

Practical Tips For Meal Planning

Meal planning takes on a nuanced significance for individuals navigating the complexities of Crohn's disease, a chronic condition impacting the gastrointestinal tract. Crafting a thoughtful approach to meals not only helps manage symptoms but also promotes overall well-being and resilience. From identifying trigger foods to ensuring adequate nutrition, the following practical tips offer guidance for individuals undertaking the journey "Beyond the Bowels" through mindful and adaptive meal planning.

1. Keep a Food Diary:
Initiate meal planning by keeping a detailed food diary. Record daily meals, snacks, and any associated symptoms. This helps identify patterns, trigger foods, and individual tolerances, forming a foundation for personalized meal plans.

2. Identify Trigger Foods:

Collaborate with healthcare providers to identify trigger foods that may exacerbate symptoms. Common triggers include high-fiber foods, spicy dishes, and certain dairy products. Avoidance or moderation of these foods can be integrated into meal planning.

3. Focus on Nutrient Density:
Prioritize nutrient-dense foods to ensure optimal nutrition. Incorporate a variety of fruits, vegetables, lean proteins, and whole grains. Nutrient-dense choices support overall health and can be tailored to individual tolerances.

4. Meal Frequency and Portion Control:
Consider smaller, more frequent meals to ease digestion and minimize discomfort. Portion control is crucial to prevent overloading the digestive system. Aim for balanced meals that include protein, healthy fats, and well-tolerated carbohydrates.

5. Cooking Methods:
Choose gentle cooking methods that preserve nutrients and ease digestion. Methods such as steaming, baking, and grilling are generally well-tolerated. Experiment with cooking techniques to identify those that suit individual preferences.

6. Experiment with Elimination Diets:
Under the guidance of healthcare providers, explore elimination diets to identify and manage

trigger foods. Gradual reintroduction of eliminated foods helps pinpoint tolerances and allows for a more varied diet.

7. Stay Hydrated:
Adequate hydration is vital for individuals with Crohn's. Include hydrating foods like soups, fruits, and vegetables in meal plans. Monitor fluid intake, especially during flare-ups, to prevent dehydration.

8. Incorporate Omega-3 Fatty Acids:
Include sources of omega-3 fatty acids, such as fatty fish or flaxseeds, known for their anti-inflammatory properties. These can contribute to managing inflammation associated with Crohn's.

9. Prep and Plan Ahead:
Simplify meal preparation by prepping ingredients in advance. Chop vegetables, marinate proteins, or batch-cook grains to streamline cooking and minimize stress during mealtime.

10. Listen to Your Body:
Pay attention to hunger and fullness cues. Listen to your body's signals and adjust meal sizes accordingly. Intuitive eating fosters a mindful approach to nourishing your body.

11. Nutritional Supplements:
In consultation with healthcare providers, consider incorporating nutritional supplements to address deficiencies or during periods of increased

nutritional needs. These can provide essential nutrients in a concentrated form.

12. Mindful Eating Practices:
Practice mindful eating to enhance the dining experience. Chew food thoroughly, savor flavors, and eat in a calm environment. Mindful practices contribute to better digestion and enjoyment of meals.

13. Explore Food Substitutions:
Experiment with food substitutions for trigger items. For instance, lactose-free dairy or gluten-free alternatives may be suitable for some individuals. Tailor meal plans to accommodate specific dietary needs.

14. Collaborate with a Dietitian:
Work closely with a registered dietitian specializing in gastrointestinal disorders. A dietitian can provide personalized guidance, create meal plans, and offer support in navigating dietary challenges associated with Crohn's.

15. Social and Emotional Considerations:
Consider social and emotional aspects when planning meals. Communicate dietary needs with friends and family to ensure a supportive dining environment. Engage in stress-reducing practices to foster a positive relationship with food.

16. Variety and Experimentation:

Embrace variety in meals to ensure a well-rounded diet. Experiment with new recipes and ingredients that align with individual tolerances. A diverse diet contributes to better overall nutrition.

Navigating meal planning with Crohn's disease requires flexibility, experimentation, and a proactive approach. By incorporating these practical tips into daily life, individuals can cultivate resilience, enjoy nourishing meals, and embark on a journey "Beyond the Bowels" that embraces the positive impact of mindful and adaptive meal planning on overall well-being.

Lifestyle Adjustment For Wellness

Embarking on the journey of managing Crohn's disease goes beyond medical interventions; it necessitates a comprehensive embrace of lifestyle adjustments that prioritize holistic wellness. In the intricate tapestry of Crohn's, where the gastrointestinal system is the focal point of challenge, lifestyle choices become integral threads weaving together physical health, emotional resilience, and a thriving spirit. This section delves into the profound impact of lifestyle adjustments on the well-being of individuals navigating Crohn's, exploring the dynamic interplay between daily choices and the journey "Beyond the Bowels." From stress management to regular physical activity, nurturing social connections, and fostering a positive mindset, these adjustments not only complement medical management but empower individuals to actively shape a life that transcends the constraints of their condition. By acknowledging the interconnectedness of lifestyle and wellness, individuals with Crohn's are guided toward a path where each choice becomes an opportunity for resilience, empowerment, and the pursuit of a vibrant and fulfilling life amidst the challenges posed by this chronic inflammatory condition.

Chapter 6

Exercise And Crohn's: Finding The Right Balance

Embarking on an exercise regimen can be a delicate yet empowering aspect of managing Crohn's disease, a chronic condition that impacts the gastrointestinal tract. The intricate relationship between physical activity and the symptoms of Crohn's requires individuals to find a nuanced balance that promotes overall well-being without exacerbating their condition. This exploration delves into the multifaceted considerations surrounding exercise and Crohn's, offering insights on the benefits, potential challenges, and strategies for finding the right balance. From the positive impact of regular physical activity on mental health to tailored approaches for individuals during flare-ups, this guide empowers those navigating the journey "Beyond the Bowels" to integrate exercise into their lives as a source of strength, resilience, and improved quality of life.

1. Understanding the Benefits:
Regular exercise has been associated with numerous health benefits, including improved mood, increased energy levels, and enhanced overall well-being. For individuals with Crohn's, the positive impact extends to potential reductions in inflammation and stress, contributing to better disease management.

2. Tailoring Exercise to Individual Needs:
Recognizing the variability in symptoms and tolerances among individuals with Crohn's, it's crucial to tailor exercise plans to individual needs. This may involve consulting with healthcare providers and fitness professionals to create personalized routines that align with overall health goals.

3. Low-Impact Activities:
Low-impact exercises, such as walking, swimming, or cycling, are often well-tolerated by individuals with Crohn's. These activities provide cardiovascular benefits without placing excessive strain on the digestive system, making them suitable options for many.

4. Strength Training and Flexibility:
Incorporating strength training and flexibility exercises can contribute to overall fitness. These activities enhance muscle tone, improve joint function, and support individuals in maintaining a strong and resilient body.

5. Monitoring Symptoms:
Close monitoring of symptoms is essential, particularly during and after exercise. Individuals should be attentive to any signs of discomfort, fatigue, or exacerbation of symptoms. Adjustments to intensity and duration may be necessary based on individual responses.

6. Timing Around Meals:
Planning exercise sessions around meals can be strategic. Waiting a sufficient amount of time after eating helps prevent digestive discomfort, while engaging in physical activity may stimulate appetite and improve digestion.

7. Hydration and Electrolyte Balance:
Maintaining proper hydration is crucial, especially considering the potential fluid losses during exercise. Ensuring an adequate balance of electrolytes supports hydration and helps prevent complications related to dehydration.

8. Stress Management Through Exercise:

Exercise serves as a potent tool for stress management, a factor known to influence Crohn's symptoms. Incorporating stress-reducing activities, such as yoga or meditation, as part of an exercise routine contributes to both mental and physical well-being.

9. Adapting During Flare-Ups:
During flare-ups or periods of increased symptoms, individuals may need to adapt their exercise routines. This could involve choosing gentler activities, reducing intensity, or focusing on flexibility and mobility exercises until symptoms subside.

10. Consultation with Healthcare Providers:
Open communication with healthcare providers is fundamental. Consulting with gastroenterologists or healthcare teams helps ensure that exercise plans align with medical management and individual health considerations.

11. Gradual Progression:
Gradual progression is key, especially for those new to exercise or reinitiating physical activity after a period of inactivity. Incremental increases in intensity and duration allow the body to adapt and minimize the risk of triggering symptoms.

12. Engaging in Social Activities:
Participating in social or group exercise activities can enhance motivation and foster a sense of

community. Engaging in activities with others provides a supportive environment and adds a social dimension to the exercise routine.

13. Embracing Variety:
Variety in exercise routines prevents monotony and allows individuals to explore activities that align with their preferences and tolerances. From outdoor activities to group classes, incorporating variety contributes to a dynamic and enjoyable fitness routine.

14. Individualized Approaches:

Every individual's response to exercise is unique. Recognizing and respecting these individual differences allows for the development of exercise plans that enhance well-being without compromising health.

15. Celebrating Achievements:
Celebrating achievements, no matter how small, contributes to a positive mindset and motivation to maintain an active lifestyle. Setting realistic goals and acknowledging progress fosters a sense of accomplishment.

Navigating the delicate balance between exercise and Crohn's disease involves a thoughtful and individualized approach. By integrating these considerations into their routines, individuals can harness the positive benefits of exercise while respecting the nuances of their condition. The journey "Beyond the Bowels" encompasses not only physical health but also the cultivation of strength, resilience, and a thriving spirit through balanced and adapted exercise routines.

Sleep, Stress And Crohn's: A Holistic Approach

Navigating the complexities of Crohn's disease demands a holistic approach that extends beyond medical interventions, delving into the intricate relationship between sleep, stress, and overall well-being. This exploration explores the profound impact of these interconnected elements on the management of Crohn's, offering insights into the bidirectional nature of their influence and strategies for fostering a harmonious balance. From the role of quality sleep in immune function to stress management techniques that complement medical care, individuals embarking on the journey "Beyond the Bowels" can cultivate resilience and optimize their health by embracing a holistic approach that recognizes the interconnected dynamics of sleep, stress, and Crohn's disease.

1. Sleep Quality and Immune Function:
Quality sleep is foundational to immune function, playing a pivotal role in the body's ability to regulate inflammation. For individuals with Crohn's, prioritizing consistent and restorative sleep becomes crucial in supporting overall health and mitigating the impact of chronic inflammation.

2. Establishing a Sleep Routine:
Creating a consistent sleep routine contributes to better sleep quality. Establishing regular sleep and wake times, creating a comfortable sleep environment, and minimizing stimulating activities before bedtime are key components of a supportive sleep routine.

3. Mind-Body Practices for Sleep:
Incorporating mind-body practices, such as meditation or relaxation techniques, promotes relaxation before bedtime. These practices contribute to stress reduction and enhance the likelihood of achieving restful sleep for individuals managing the challenges of Crohn's.

4. Addressing Sleep Disruptions:
Individuals with Crohn's may experience sleep disruptions due to symptoms, medication side

effects, or stress. Collaborating with healthcare providers to address underlying causes and exploring strategies to manage these disruptions is essential for restoring healthy sleep patterns.

5. The Impact of Stress on Crohn's:
Stress has been identified as a potential trigger for Crohn's flares and an exacerbating factor for symptoms. A holistic approach involves adopting stress management techniques to minimize the impact of stress on both physical and mental well-being.

6. Stress-Reduction Techniques:
Engaging in stress-reduction techniques, such as deep breathing exercises, mindfulness, or yoga, fosters a resilient response to stressors. Regular practice of these techniques provides individuals with tools to navigate the emotional complexities associated with Crohn's.

7. Physical Activity and Stress Reduction:
Regular physical activity serves as a dual-purpose tool, contributing to both stress reduction and overall well-being. Tailored exercise routines that align with individual tolerances can be incorporated into a holistic approach to managing stress.

8. Cognitive Behavioral Therapy (CBT):
CBT is a therapeutic approach that addresses the relationship between thoughts, feelings, and behaviors. It has shown efficacy in managing stress

and improving coping mechanisms, making it a valuable tool for individuals navigating the emotional landscape of Crohn's.

9. Nutrition and Stress Resilience:
Recognizing the connection between nutrition and stress resilience is essential. A well-balanced diet that includes nutrient-dense foods contributes not only to physical health but also to the body's ability to manage stress more effectively.

10. Social Support and Coping Strategies:
Cultivating social support networks and employing effective coping strategies are integral components of a holistic approach. Sharing experiences, seeking support from loved ones, and connecting with communities that understand the challenges of Crohn's contribute to emotional well-being.

11. Professional Mental Health Support:
Seeking professional mental health support, such as counseling or therapy, is a proactive step in managing stress associated with Crohn's. Mental health professionals provide tools for coping, strategies for stress management, and a safe space for exploring and processing emotions.

12. Biofeedback and Relaxation Techniques:
Biofeedback and relaxation techniques provide individuals with tangible tools for managing stress responses. These approaches allow for the conscious regulation of physiological processes,

fostering a sense of control over the body's reactions to stressors.

13. Sleep Hygiene and Lifestyle Adjustments: Embracing sleep hygiene practices, such as limiting screen time before bed and creating a conducive sleep environment, enhances the quality of sleep. Lifestyle adjustments that support overall well-being, such as regular physical activity and a balanced diet, contribute to better sleep and stress management.

14. Hydration and Nutrition for Resilience: Adequate hydration and proper nutrition contribute to resilience in the face of stress. Maintaining optimal hydration levels and nourishing the body with nutrient-dense foods provide a foundation for both physical and emotional well-being.

15. Individualized Approaches to Holistic Health: Recognizing the uniqueness of each individual's experience with Crohn's disease, a holistic approach encourages personalized strategies. Tailoring sleep routines, stress management techniques, and lifestyle adjustments to align with individual needs fosters a more effective and sustainable approach to overall well-being.

By embracing a holistic approach that integrates quality sleep, stress management, and individualized strategies into the management of Crohn's disease, individuals can foster resilience, optimize their health, and embark on a journey "Beyond the Bowels" that encompasses not only physical wellness but also emotional strength and a thriving spirit despite the challenges posed by Crohn's disease.

Balancing Work And Personal Life

Managing the intricacies of work and personal life can pose unique challenges for individuals grappling with Crohn's disease. This chronic inflammatory condition, primarily affecting the gastrointestinal tract, requires a delicate balance to ensure both professional success and personal well-being. This exploration delves into the multifaceted aspects of navigating the intersection of work and personal life with Crohn's, offering insights into strategies for maintaining productivity, fostering understanding in the workplace, and prioritizing self-care in the pursuit of a harmonious and fulfilling life "Beyond the Bowels."

1. Open Communication in the Workplace:
Establishing open communication with employers and colleagues is paramount. Sharing insights about Crohn's, including potential challenges and necessary accommodations, fosters understanding and creates a supportive work environment.

2. Flexible Work Arrangements:
Exploring flexible work arrangements, such as remote work or adjusted hours, can provide individuals with Crohn's the flexibility needed to manage symptoms and navigate the unpredictable nature of the condition.

3. Prioritizing Self-Care:
Prioritizing self-care is essential for individuals with Crohn's. This involves recognizing personal limits, setting boundaries, and scheduling regular breaks to manage stress and maintain overall well-being.

4. Effective Time Management:
Implementing effective time management strategies is crucial. Prioritizing tasks, breaking them into manageable steps, and establishing realistic deadlines contribute to maintaining productivity while minimizing stress.

5. Building a Supportive Network:
Cultivating a supportive network within the workplace and personal life is invaluable. Having colleagues, friends, and family members who understand and empathize with the challenges of Crohn's enhances emotional well-being and provides a safety net during challenging times.

6. Utilizing Accommodations:
Employing reasonable accommodations, such as ergonomic workspace adjustments or access to private restroom facilities, ensures that the workplace is conducive to the needs of individuals with Crohn's.

7. Managing Stress in the Workplace:
Adopting stress management techniques is crucial for maintaining balance. Techniques such as deep breathing exercises, mindfulness, or short breaks during the workday contribute to managing stressors associated with both work and Crohn's.

8. Strategic Meal Planning:
Strategic meal planning in the workplace involves considering dietary needs and planning meals that align with individual tolerances. Bringing nutritious snacks and meals to work ensures that individuals with Crohn's can maintain energy levels and manage symptoms effectively.

9. Advocacy for Work-Life Balance:

Advocating for work-life balance is a proactive step. Encouraging a workplace culture that values well-being, respects personal boundaries, and understands the importance of a balanced life contributes to the overall health and satisfaction of employees with Crohn's.

10. Utilizing Sick Leave Appropriately:
Recognizing the importance of utilizing sick leave when needed is crucial. Taking time off to manage flare-ups or attend medical appointments allows individuals to prioritize health without compromising their professional responsibilities.

11. Remote Work Considerations:
Remote work considerations, when feasible, offer individuals with Crohn's the opportunity to work in an environment that is comfortable and accommodates their specific needs, reducing the impact of commuting and office-related stressors.

12. Balancing Social and Professional Obligations:
Striking a balance between social and professional obligations is key. While networking and professional engagements are important, ensuring that these activities align with energy levels and symptom management prevents burnout.

13. Embracing Flexibility:
Embracing flexibility in both work and personal life allows individuals to adapt to the dynamic nature of Crohn's disease. This includes being open to

adjusting plans based on symptom fluctuations and recognizing that flexibility is a strength.

14. Setting Realistic Goals:
Setting realistic and achievable goals, both in the workplace and personal life, prevents undue stress and promotes a sense of accomplishment. Breaking down larger tasks into smaller, manageable steps facilitates a proactive approach to achieving objectives.

15. Professional Development and Growth:
Investing in professional development and growth while considering individual health needs is crucial. Balancing career aspirations with the requirements of Crohn's involves strategic planning and a focus on achievable milestones.

16. Regular Health Check-Ins:
Regular health check-ins with healthcare providers ensure that individuals with Crohn's are proactively managing their health. This allows for timely adjustments to medical management and helps prevent potential setbacks in both work and personal life.

Navigating the delicate balance between work and personal life with Crohn's disease requires adaptability, effective communication, and a commitment to self-care. By integrating these strategies into their daily lives, individuals can cultivate resilience, maintain professional success, and embark on a fulfilling journey "Beyond the Bowels" that embraces both career aspirations and holistic well-being.

Family And Relationship

Crohn's disease, with its complex tapestry of symptoms and uncertainties, not only impacts the individual bearing its weight but also ripples through the fabric of family and relationships. This introductory exploration delves into the profound interplay between Crohn's and the bonds that tie us together, recognizing that the support and understanding of loved ones are integral to the journey "Beyond the Bowels." Families are thrust into a dynamic landscape where empathy, patience, and resilience become essential tools. Relationships, both romantic and platonic, undergo a metamorphosis as they navigate the highs and lows of living with a chronic inflammatory condition. This section examines not only the challenges that may arise but also the potential for growth, understanding, and unity within the framework of family and relationships. By fostering open communication, embracing flexibility, and cultivating a shared commitment to well-being, individuals with Crohn's, along with their loved ones, can embark on a collective journey that transcends the limitations imposed by the disease, weaving a narrative of strength, compassion, and unity in the face of adversity.

Chapter 7

Communicating About Crohn's With Loved Ones

Engaging in open and honest communication about Crohn's disease with loved ones is a pivotal aspect of the journey "Beyond the Bowels." This chronic inflammatory condition, with its unpredictable nature, demands a shared understanding within relationships to foster support, empathy, and resilience. This exploration delves into the intricacies of communicating about Crohn's, providing insights into initiating conversations, addressing emotions, and building a foundation of mutual understanding that strengthens familial and interpersonal bonds.

1. Initiating the Conversation:
Starting the conversation about Crohn's requires a thoughtful and considerate approach. Choosing a calm and private setting allows for focused dialogue, creating an atmosphere conducive to open communication.

2. Educating Loved Ones:
Providing educational resources or accompanying loved ones to medical appointments can be instrumental in conveying essential information about Crohn's disease. Understanding the basics,

such as symptoms, treatment options, and potential challenges, equips loved ones with the knowledge needed to offer meaningful support.

3. Expressing Emotions:
Encouraging the expression of emotions is vital. Both individuals with Crohn's and their loved ones may experience a range of feelings, from fear and frustration to empathy and concern. Acknowledging and validating these emotions fosters a safe space for open dialogue.

4. Sharing Personal Experiences:
Personal narratives hold immense power in bridging understanding. Sharing individual experiences with Crohn's, including challenges and triumphs, offers loved ones a glimpse into the daily realities of living with the condition and cultivates empathy.

5. Setting Realistic Expectations:
Establishing realistic expectations is key to navigating the impact of Crohn's on relationships. Communicating openly about potential fluctuations in health, energy levels, and the need for flexibility sets the groundwork for understanding the nuances of the condition.

6. Encouraging Questions and Dialogue:
Creating an environment where questions are welcome encourages ongoing dialogue. Loved ones may have inquiries about the condition,

treatment plans, or ways to provide support. Fostering an atmosphere of openness paves the way for continued communication.

7. Discussing Practical Needs:
Practical needs, such as dietary considerations, medication routines, and potential lifestyle adjustments, are integral components of the conversation. Addressing these aspects ensures that loved ones are well-informed and can actively participate in supporting the individual with Crohn's.

8. Building a Support System:
Emphasizing the importance of a support system is crucial. Discussing the roles that various individuals, including friends, family, and healthcare providers, can play in the support network reinforces the idea that navigating Crohn's is a collective effort.

9. Addressing Concerns and Fears:
Loved ones may harbor concerns and fears about the impact of Crohn's on the individual's health and the dynamics of the relationship. Creating space for these concerns and addressing them openly contributes to building trust and understanding.

10. Celebrating Milestones and Victories:
Acknowledging and celebrating milestones and victories, no matter how small, strengthens the narrative of resilience. Sharing successes in managing symptoms or overcoming challenges

reinforces the collective journey of triumph over adversity.

11. Encouraging Empathy and Patience:
Encouraging empathy and patience within relationships is an ongoing process. Reminding loved ones that the impact of Crohn's may vary day to day fosters a culture of understanding and adaptability.

12. Collaborative Decision-Making:
Involving loved ones in collaborative decision-making, especially regarding treatment plans or adjustments to daily routines, fosters a sense of shared responsibility. This approach reinforces that navigating Crohn's is a team effort.

13. Respecting Boundaries:
Respecting individual boundaries is essential. Loved ones should be aware that there may be times when individuals with Crohn's need space or time for self-care. Establishing and respecting these boundaries contributes to overall well-being.

14. Reassurance and Affirmation:
Providing reassurance and affirmation reinforces the importance of emotional support. Reminding loved ones that their understanding and presence are valued contributes to a sense of security within the relationship.

15. Ongoing Communication:

Ongoing communication is a cornerstone of navigating Crohn's within relationships. Regular check-ins, updates on health status, and a continuous dialogue about evolving needs and expectations ensure that the lines of communication remain open and adaptive.

Navigating conversations about Crohn's with loved ones requires patience, empathy, and a commitment to shared understanding. By embracing open dialogue and fostering an environment of support, individuals with Crohn's and their loved ones can embark on a journey that strengthens bonds, nurtures resilience, and transcends the challenges posed by this chronic inflammatory condition.

Building Stronger Relationships

The journey with Crohn's disease is not solitary; it intertwines with the fabric of relationships, presenting opportunities for growth, understanding, and resilience. Building stronger connections amidst the challenges of Crohn's requires intention, communication, and a shared commitment to navigating the complexities "Beyond the Bowels." This exploration delves into strategies and insights aimed at fortifying relationships—both familial and interpersonal—nurturing an environment where empathy, flexibility, and unwavering support create a foundation for enduring and thriving relationships.

1. Open and Honest Communication:
The bedrock of any strong relationship lies in open and honest communication. For individuals with Crohn's, expressing needs, sharing experiences, and discussing challenges openly fosters a climate of understanding and empathy.

2. Educating Loved Ones:
Knowledge is a powerful tool in fostering understanding. Providing educational materials or attending medical appointments together equips loved ones with the information needed to comprehend the intricacies of Crohn's and actively participate in the journey.

3. Cultivating Empathy:
Cultivating empathy involves actively seeking to understand the perspective of the individual with Crohn's. Putting oneself in their shoes and recognizing the emotional and physical toll of the

condition builds a deeper connection and mutual compassion.

4. Mutual Goal Setting:
Setting mutual goals creates a shared sense of purpose. Whether it's crafting lifestyle adjustments, supporting treatment plans, or prioritizing self-care, collaborating on common objectives strengthens the sense of partnership in navigating Crohn's.

5. Navigating Lifestyle Adjustments Together:
The impact of Crohn's often necessitates lifestyle adjustments. Facing these changes as a team, whether related to diet, exercise, or daily routines, ensures that both individuals are actively involved and supportive of the adaptations required.

6. Building a Support Network:
The broader support network, including friends, family, and healthcare professionals, plays a pivotal role. Actively involving loved ones in this network reinforces that managing Crohn's is a collective effort, distributing the emotional and practical load.

7. Prioritizing Quality Time:
Quality time becomes a cherished currency in relationships affected by chronic illness. Prioritizing moments of connection, whether through shared activities or simple gestures, reinforces the bond and offers respite from the challenges of Crohn's.

8. Expressing Gratitude:
Expressing gratitude for the support and understanding offered creates a positive and affirming atmosphere. Recognizing and acknowledging the efforts made by loved ones fosters a sense of mutual appreciation.

9. Adaptability and Flexibility:
The unpredictable nature of Crohn's demands adaptability and flexibility. Embracing change with resilience and a sense of humor fortifies relationships, allowing both individuals to navigate the uncertainties together.

10. Shared Coping Strategies:
Coping with the emotional aspects of Crohn's involves shared strategies. Whether engaging in stress-reducing activities, practicing mindfulness together, or seeking professional support as a team, shared coping mechanisms enhance resilience.

11. Celebrating Milestones:
Celebrating milestones, whether related to health achievements or personal victories, contributes to a positive and supportive environment. Recognizing progress reinforces the narrative of resilience and shared triumphs over the challenges posed by Crohn's.

12. Maintaining Intimacy:

Nurturing intimacy is essential in relationships impacted by chronic illness. Communicating openly about emotional and physical needs, expressing affection, and prioritizing intimacy contribute to the overall well-being of the partnership.

13. Respecting Individual Boundaries:
Recognizing and respecting individual boundaries is a cornerstone of a healthy relationship. Understanding when to offer support and when to provide space cultivates a sense of autonomy and consideration for each other's needs.

14. Weathering Flare-Ups Together:
Flare-ups are an inevitable part of the Crohn's journey. Navigating these challenging periods together, offering unwavering support, and adapting plans as needed reinforce the resilience of the relationship.

15. Seeking Professional Support:
Recognizing when professional support is needed is a proactive step. Seeking couples counseling or therapy provides a safe space to address challenges, enhance communication skills, and fortify the relationship's foundation.

16. Continuous Check-Ins:
Regular check-ins ensure that the lines of communication remain open. A continuous dialogue about evolving needs, emotions, and expectations strengthens the relationship's

adaptability and responsiveness to the dynamics of Crohn's.

Building stronger relationships amidst the complexities of Crohn's disease involves a shared commitment to understanding, flexibility, and mutual support. By actively engaging in these strategies, individuals and their loved ones can fortify the bonds that transcend the challenges posed by chronic illness, fostering relationships that not only endure but thrive "Beyond the Bowels."

parenting with crohn's: challenges and triumphs

Parenting is a profound journey filled with challenges and triumphs, and when intertwined with the complexities of Crohn's disease, it becomes a unique terrain that demands resilience, adaptability, and unwavering determination. This exploration delves into the multifaceted aspects of parenting with Crohn's, shedding light on the trials faced by individuals managing both the responsibilities of parenthood and the unpredictable nature of this chronic inflammatory condition. From the early stages of family planning to the day-to-day joys and hurdles of raising children, this discussion encapsulates the challenges and triumphs, offering insights into strategies that empower parents with Crohn's to navigate this intricate path while celebrating the resilience and strength that parenthood can bring.

1. Family Planning Considerations:
The journey of parenting with Crohn's often begins with considerations about family planning. Individuals with Crohn's may navigate conversations with healthcare providers to ensure a proactive and informed approach to managing the condition during pregnancy and childbirth.

2. Navigating Pregnancy:
Pregnancy introduces a unique set of considerations for individuals with Crohn's. Collaborating closely with healthcare teams to manage symptoms, adjust medications, and address potential complications becomes pivotal, ensuring the health and well-being of both the parent and the baby.

3. Balancing Parenthood and Fluctuating Symptoms:
Parenthood unfolds amidst the backdrop of fluctuating Crohn's symptoms. The challenge lies in striking a balance between meeting the needs of children while managing the unpredictable nature of the condition. Strategies involve effective time management, communication with family members, and prioritizing self-care.

4. Managing Energy Levels and Fatigue:
Crohn's symptoms, such as fatigue, can impact energy levels. Parents with Crohn's must navigate the delicate balance of allocating energy to parenting responsibilities while ensuring self-preservation. Prioritizing tasks, seeking support, and practicing self-compassion become crucial elements.

5. Building a Support Network:
A robust support network is instrumental in parenting with Crohn's. Cultivating relationships with family, friends, and other parents provides a safety net of assistance during challenging times and contributes to a sense of community.

6. Addressing the Emotional Toll:
The emotional toll of Crohn's can intersect with the emotional demands of parenting. Open communication with a partner, seeking counseling or support groups, and acknowledging emotions contribute to maintaining emotional well-being within the family dynamic.

7. Incorporating Children in Self-Care Practices:
Parenting with Crohn's involves not only caring for children but also modeling self-care practices. Involving children in age-appropriate discussions about health, teaching them the importance of empathy, and fostering a collaborative approach to family well-being are key elements.

8. Adapting to Unpredictable Schedules:
Crohn's symptoms often follow an unpredictable schedule. Adapting to these uncertainties requires flexibility in parenting routines. Establishing backup plans, communicating with children about potential changes, and cultivating adaptability within the family dynamic contribute to a harmonious environment.

9. Prioritizing Quality Time:
Prioritizing quality time with children becomes an anchor in the face of life's uncertainties. Focusing on meaningful interactions, shared activities, and creating positive memories contribute to the emotional resilience of both parents and children.

10. Teaching Resilience and Empathy:
Parenting with Crohn's offers an opportunity to teach children valuable life skills. Instilling resilience, empathy, and adaptability through age-appropriate conversations about health challenges fosters a supportive family culture.

11. Celebrating Parenting Milestones:
Celebrating parenting milestones, both big and small, contributes to a positive family dynamic. Acknowledging achievements, overcoming challenges, and collectively celebrating the journey foster a sense of unity and accomplishment.

12. Parental Self-Advocacy:

Advocating for oneself as a parent with Crohn's is crucial. This involves clear communication with healthcare providers, asserting needs within the family structure, and recognizing when additional support or adjustments are necessary.

13. Planning for Childcare During Flare-Ups:
Flare-ups may necessitate temporary adjustments in childcare responsibilities. Planning ahead for these situations, whether through a support network, extended family, or professional assistance, ensures that children are cared for during periods of increased health challenges.

14. Seeking Professional Guidance:
Seeking professional guidance, such as counseling or family therapy, provides a space for open communication and support. Professional intervention can offer coping strategies, facilitate discussions, and enhance the overall resilience of the family unit.

15. Encouraging Independence in Children:
Fostering independence in children is a pivotal aspect of parenting with Crohn's. Encouraging age-appropriate responsibilities, open communication about health, and empowering children to contribute to the family's well-being contribute to a collaborative family environment.

Parenting with Crohn's is a transformative journey that encompasses both challenges and triumphs.

By embracing proactive communication, building a supportive network, and prioritizing both individual and family well-being, parents with Crohn's can navigate the intricacies of parenthood while celebrating the joys and resilience that this journey brings "Beyond the Bowels."

Thriving Despite Crohn's Disease

In the realm of chronic illness, the narrative often tends to focus on the challenges and limitations, overshadowing the remarkable stories of resilience and triumph that unfold in the face of adversity. Within the landscape of Crohn's disease, a condition characterized by its unpredictable nature and profound impact on daily life, there exists a narrative of strength, tenacity, and unwavering determination. This exploration delves into the concept of not merely surviving but thriving despite Crohn's disease, illuminating the myriad ways individuals navigate the complexities of their health while embracing a life that extends far beyond the confines of their diagnosis. From the initial steps of understanding the condition to cultivating a holistic approach that encompasses physical, emotional, and social well-being, this journey is a testament to the indomitable spirit that propels individuals to not only endure but to flourish despite the challenges posed by Crohn's. By weaving together stories of resilience, insights into self-care practices, and a celebration of personal victories, this exploration embarks on a path that transcends the limitations of chronic illness, inspiring individuals to embark on a journey of thriving "Beyond the Bowels."

Chapter 8

Success Stories: Inspiring Journeys

Amidst the tumultuous terrain of Crohn's disease, there emerges a tapestry of inspiring success stories, each thread woven with resilience, courage, and the unwavering spirit to transcend the limitations imposed by chronic illness. These narratives defy the conventional expectations associated with health challenges, offering glimpses into the extraordinary journeys of individuals who have not merely navigated the complexities of Crohn's but have emerged as beacons of hope and inspiration. From embracing a holistic approach to well-being to achieving milestones that extend far beyond medical prognoses, these success stories illuminate the indomitable human spirit. This exploration delves into the diverse and uplifting tales of those who have turned the page on despair, illustrating that a life filled with purpose, achievements, and joy is not only possible but is being actively pursued by individuals thriving amidst the challenges posed by Crohn's disease. Through tales of personal victories, community support, and a commitment to holistic health, these stories transcend the narrative of illness, offering a powerful testament to the potential for triumph despite the formidable presence of Crohn's. By shining a spotlight on these inspiring journeys, we celebrate the resilience that propels individuals to not only confront but conquer the hurdles on their path, painting a vivid picture of success and empowerment that echoes "Beyond the Bowels."

Setting Goals And Pursuing Dreams

The journey with Crohn's disease introduces a unique set of challenges, but it does not diminish the power of dreams or the ability to set and achieve meaningful goals. In fact, individuals navigating the complexities of Crohn's often exemplify unparalleled resilience and determination as they pursue their aspirations. This exploration delves into the art of goal-setting and dream pursuit within the context of Crohn's disease, highlighting the strategies, mindset shifts, and community support that empower individuals to not only face their health challenges but to actively shape a future filled with accomplishments, purpose, and fulfillment.

1. Mindset Shifts:
The foundation of pursuing dreams with Crohn's lies in cultivating a resilient mindset. Shifting from a perspective of limitations to one of possibilities enables individuals to approach their goals with creativity, adaptability, and a determination to overcome obstacles.

2. Setting Realistic and Adaptive Goals:
Goal-setting involves a delicate balance between ambition and realism. Individuals with Crohn's benefit from setting goals that align with their health needs, allowing for adaptability to accommodate the unpredictable nature of the condition.

3. Breaking Down Goals into Manageable Steps:
Breaking down larger goals into manageable steps is a key strategy. This approach not only makes aspirations more achievable but also allows for better navigation of energy levels, symptom fluctuations, and the day-to-day demands of managing Crohn's.

4. Utilizing Support Systems:
Building a robust support system is instrumental in goal pursuit. Whether through healthcare providers, friends, family, or communities that understand the challenges of Crohn's, having a network that

provides encouragement, understanding, and practical assistance is invaluable.

5. Prioritizing Self-Care:
Goal pursuit is most effective when rooted in a foundation of self-care. Prioritizing physical, emotional, and mental well-being ensures that individuals have the resilience and energy required to actively engage in the pursuit of their dreams.

6. Flexible Planning:
Recognizing the need for flexibility in planning is crucial. Individuals with Crohn's may encounter unexpected health challenges, and being adaptable in adjusting timelines or approaches to goals is a strength that enhances the likelihood of success.

7. Celebrating Small Victories:
Celebrating small victories along the way contributes to a positive and motivating journey. Recognizing and acknowledging progress, no matter how incremental, fosters a sense of achievement and sustains momentum.

8. Inspiring and Learning from Others:
Drawing inspiration from others who have navigated similar journeys is empowering. Learning from their experiences, understanding their strategies, and realizing the potential for success despite Crohn's fosters a sense of community and shared achievement.

9. Incorporating Passion and Purpose:
Pursuing dreams is most fulfilling when rooted in passion and purpose. Identifying what truly matters and aligning goals with personal values enhances motivation, making the journey with Crohn's not only purposeful but deeply meaningful.

10. Utilizing Professional Guidance:
Seeking guidance from professionals, such as career counselors, life coaches, or healthcare providers, adds a layer of expertise to goal-setting. These professionals can offer insights, strategies, and support tailored to the unique challenges associated with Crohn's.

11. Embracing Resilience in Setbacks:
Setbacks are a natural part of any journey, and embracing resilience in the face of setbacks is crucial. Individuals with Crohn's learn to navigate setbacks with a sense of adaptability, learning, and the determination to persist in their pursuit of dreams.

12. Building a Holistic Vision of Success:
Success, in the context of Crohn's, extends beyond traditional definitions. Building a holistic vision of success that encompasses well-being, personal growth, and meaningful connections ensures that individuals derive fulfillment from their pursuits.

13. Advocating for Accommodations:

Advocating for accommodations when necessary is an important aspect of goal pursuit with Crohn's. Whether in the workplace, academic settings, or personal endeavors, ensuring that environments support health needs contributes to sustained success.

14. Reflecting and Adjusting Goals:
Periodic reflection and adjustment of goals is a dynamic and empowering process. Individuals with Crohn's learn to reassess their aspirations, adapting them to align with evolving circumstances and ensuring that the pursuit of dreams remains a positive and realistic endeavor.

15. Creating a Legacy of Inspiration:
The pursuit of dreams with Crohn's has the power to inspire others. Creating a legacy of inspiration involves sharing one's journey, offering insights, and showcasing the possibilities for success despite the challenges posed by chronic illness.

Pursuing dreams with Crohn's disease is not a mere aspiration; it is a testament to the extraordinary resilience and strength that individuals possess. By embracing adaptive strategies, fostering a resilient mindset, and seeking support, individuals with Crohn's can actively shape a future that not only acknowledges their health challenges but also celebrates the boundless potential for achievement "Beyond the Bowels."

Finding Joy And Purpose

In the intricate tapestry of living with Crohn's disease, discovering joy and purpose becomes a transformative journey that transcends the boundaries of health challenges. This exploration delves into the art of cultivating a life rich in fulfillment and meaning, despite the presence of Crohn's. From navigating the emotional landscape to fostering a mindset rooted in resilience, individuals embark on a quest that uncovers the radiant threads of joy and purpose woven into the fabric of their existence. Through community connections, embracing passions, and aligning with personal values, this exploration illuminates the myriad pathways that lead to a life that not only acknowledges the complexities of Crohn's but also radiates with the brilliance of joy and purpose.

1. Embracing Emotional Resilience:
The journey toward joy and purpose begins with embracing emotional resilience. Individuals with Crohn's learn to navigate the emotional ups and downs of living with a chronic condition, developing a robust emotional foundation that forms the cornerstone of a fulfilling life.

2. Aligning with Personal Values:
Aligning daily choices and pursuits with personal values provides a compass for navigating life with Crohn's. When actions and decisions resonate with core values, a sense of purpose emerges, contributing to a life that feels authentic and meaningful.

3. Community Connection and Support:
Building connections within a community of individuals who share similar experiences creates a sense of belonging and support. Through mutual understanding and shared insights, individuals find solace, encouragement, and the affirmation that they are not alone in their journey.

4. Fostering Meaningful Relationships:
Cultivating meaningful relationships with family, friends, and a supportive network is integral to finding joy and purpose. These connections provide emotional sustenance and create a framework for shared experiences, laughter, and mutual growth.

5. Engaging in Passionate Pursuits:
Engaging in activities that ignite passion and enthusiasm adds vibrancy to life with Crohn's. Pursuing hobbies, creative endeavors, or career paths that bring joy creates a sense of purpose and fulfillment, offering a respite from the challenges of the condition.

6. Mindfulness and Present Living:
Practicing mindfulness and present living allows individuals to savor the beauty of each moment. By immersing themselves in the present, individuals with Crohn's cultivate gratitude, resilience, and an appreciation for the joys that can be found even in the midst of health challenges.

7. Setting Realistic Goals:
Setting realistic and achievable goals aligns with the principle of finding purpose. Individuals learn to establish milestones that honor their health needs while offering a sense of accomplishment and motivation for continued growth.

8. Cultivating a Positive Mindset:
A positive mindset becomes a guiding force in the pursuit of joy and purpose. Despite the challenges of Crohn's, individuals focus on the possibilities, cultivating resilience, and viewing setbacks as opportunities for growth rather than insurmountable obstacles.

9. Advocating for Self-Care:
Advocating for self-care is paramount in the journey toward joy and purpose. Prioritizing physical, emotional, and mental well-being ensures that individuals have the energy and vitality to engage in activities that bring fulfillment and happiness.

10. Creative Expression and Outlet:

Creative expression serves as a powerful outlet for individuals with Crohn's. Whether through art, writing, or other forms of self-expression, individuals discover avenues to channel their experiences, emotions, and aspirations, creating a tangible reflection of their journey.

11. Educating and Inspiring Others:
Educating and inspiring others becomes a meaningful endeavor. Sharing one's journey, insights, and triumphs not only contributes to a sense of purpose but also empowers and uplifts others who may be navigating similar challenges.

12. Celebrating Personal Achievements:
Celebrating personal achievements, no matter how small, contributes to a positive narrative. Individuals acknowledge their resilience, courage, and growth, fostering a self-affirming perspective that fuels the pursuit of further joy and purpose.

13. Balancing Health Needs:
Finding joy and purpose involves a delicate balance with health needs. Individuals learn to listen to their bodies, adapt activities to align with energy levels, and prioritize self-care without compromising the pursuit of a meaningful and fulfilling life.

14. Exploring New Perspectives:
Exploring new perspectives and opportunities becomes a dynamic aspect of the journey. Individuals with Crohn's remain open to discovering

fresh possibilities, embracing change, and adapting their outlook to accommodate evolving aspirations and sources of joy.

15. Contributing to Causes and Community:
Contributing to causes and community efforts creates a sense of purpose beyond individual pursuits. By making a positive impact in the lives of others or championing causes that resonate, individuals with Crohn's weave their experiences into a larger tapestry of shared purpose.

16. Reflecting on Personal Growth:
Reflecting on personal growth becomes a reflective practice. Individuals acknowledge their evolution, the lessons learned from navigating Crohn's, and the resilience gained, fostering a deep appreciation for the transformative journey they have undertaken.

In the face of Crohn's disease, individuals unearth the profound capacity to discover joy and purpose, crafting a narrative that transcends the boundaries of health challenges. Through resilience, community, self-care, and the pursuit of passions, individuals with Crohn's not only navigate their condition but actively thrive, illuminating a path of fulfillment and radiance "Beyond the Bowels."

Advocacy And Community Engagement

The journey with Crohn's disease extends beyond the individual, weaving a narrative of collective strength, shared understanding, and the power of unified voices. This exploration delves into the profound impact of advocacy and community engagement within the context of Crohn's, illuminating the transformative potential when individuals, caregivers, and allies come together to raise awareness, foster support networks, and drive change. In the face of the complexities that Crohn's presents, advocacy becomes a beacon, shedding light on the challenges, triumphs, and unmet needs within the broader community. Community engagement emerges as a dynamic force, forging connections that offer empathy, shared wisdom, and a collective resolve to navigate the intricacies of living with a chronic inflammatory condition. From grassroots initiatives to global movements, this exploration celebrates the resilience embedded in advocacy and community engagement, showcasing the strength that flourishes when individuals unite to amplify their voices, challenge stigmas, and actively contribute to a landscape of understanding, support, and empowerment. Together, these endeavors create a tapestry of shared experiences, fortifying the resolve to not only endure but to thrive "Beyond the Bowels," where advocacy and community engagement become pillars of strength, solidarity, and change.

www.ingramcontent.com/pod-product-compliance
Lightning Source LLC
Chambersburg PA
CBHW070735250726
48662CB00004B/1554